# Her Loving Gift

*By*
*R. Rosalie Krizan*

# Table of Contents

# Dedication

To her parents, Richard and Christina Krizan.

# Acknowledgement

Dr. Martin Hoffman, MD-Pediatrician

Dr. David Bradley, MD - Pediatrician at U of M

Dr. Robin Fountain-Dommer, MD

Shelly Greene - at the time, she was a tech in the ICU. Every time I needed encouragement, she would play worship music on her phone, and we would praise Papa God together in the ICU.

Dr. Francis Pagani - surgeon

Dr. Jonathan Haft - surgeon

Dr. Matthew Konerman, MD

Her Husband, Austin Billings, and many others.

# About the Author

Rosalie never let her Congenital Heart Defect (or CHD for short) get in her way of living life. When she wanted to do something extraordinary, and it was within her means, she did it. Still does! At a young age, she started Taekwondo and got all the way up to a blue belt. Now, as an adult, she hopes to return one day. In Middle school, she joined the cheer squad and loved every moment of it. This is where her passion for football started. Also, in middle school, she joined the school band and played clarinet. She loved band so much that she continued that through High School. Even learned to march and did marching band all four years. She graduated from high school in May of 2014. In January of 2015, she did Community College and worked full-time. Her English classes quickly became her favorite. Not only did she graduate once, but twice! In 2017, she graduated with her American Sign Language Certificate of Completion, and in 2019, she graduated again with her Associate's degree in American English Literature of the Arts! In 2018, she went to an animal rescue center, and little did she know that same day, she found her fur-child Riley! In 2020, She met a man on Okcupid, and in May of 2021 (exactly a year after meeting in person), she married her now husband, Austin Billings.

# In the Beginning

Each and every year, there is approximately one in every one hundred children born with some form of Congenital Heart Disease. CHD for short. I happened to be one of those children.

I was born in the middle of the 90's. Hot summer Tuesday morning. I am my parents' first child. A child that they had prayed for seven years. All of my mother's scans had come back with me being a healthy baby girl. I left the hospital with my parents a few days later and started life as a Krizan. I had a hard time growing and eating at first, but everyone my mother had talked to said it was normal for a while. Then, at six months old, I was having my normal doctor baby appointments when my doctor at the time listened to my heart and discovered a small murmur. He suggested that I be taken to the hospital and get it checked right away. Through many tests, doctors and nurses discovered I had a hole in my heart and one very long valve across my heart instead of having two separate heart valves. This defect, my parents learned later, was called Atrioventricular Septal Defect, or AVSD for short. This needed to be fixed if there was any chance I was going to have life. Doctors were surprised I was even still breathing at six months old. At eight months old, on Valentine's Day, I had my first open heart surgery. My surgeon took the little pieces I had of the valves and made me a Mitral heart valve. It was not perfect, but it was sturdy. It would last me twenty-four full years of life.

# The Young Years

At the age of seven, I was going to my grandparents' church. I was in Sunday school on Easter Sunday, and my teacher was talking about Jesus. How he died for our sins because he loves us so much, but he is no longer dead but alive, and he can live inside us. It was explained to me that everyone has a spiritual hole in their hearts, and people try to fill it with earthly things, but only God can come in and fix the hole and heal it. Even at seven, I knew I had a physical hole in my heart, and I had surgery to repair my broken heart. My teacher then pulled me aside and asked if I wanted my spiritual hole fixed, too. With a nod, she pulled a chair up, pulled me into a corner, and we sat and talked. Then we prayed. I asked Jesus in my heart that day.

## School Days

As I got older, I knew I was different; I knew I always had some type of heart problem. Every year, I had to go for checkups to make sure my heart was still as healthy as it could be for my condition. In school, I always hated gym class. I would try to run, play games, play sports, or climb, but I always struggled. I hated recess; I hated feeling alone. I had a hard time making friends. My first friend, I met in the second grade. She was my bully at first, but my young self knew I should be praying for her and trying to understand where she was coming from. As the year went on, we talked and, in fact, became friends. The only elementary years I really remember, kindergarten and second grade, were my favorite. I struggled in third grade, and upon my parents' request, I got held back in third grade. In fourth grade, I was a bigger child, and I did not bring the healthiest snacks to school. My teacher pulled me out in the hallway and told me I should bring in healthier snacks because they would be better for my heart. In fifth grade, I remember my teacher's name and the wall that opened up and went into another classroom. We were one big class and had two teachers when the wall was open.

I was always a bit confused about why I needed yearly checkups because my heart was fine, and in my head, it was going to stay that way for the rest of my life.

## Middle School

Middle school and my heart got along just fine, most of the time. Middle school gym class became a problem. My heart was stable and doing really well for my condition, so of course, my doctors said that I could do gym class with no restrictions, but if I felt weird, I needed to sit down, get water, and take a break. The first new challenge was changing from regular school clothes to gym class clothes. The stalls were full of girls changing, and time was running out. The class was going to start soon, and I had not changed yet. Girls just started changing. So, I followed and started to change. This was the first time I had ever changed in front of people. No one was looking at me, right? Wrong. I was putting my gym shirt on, and a girl came up to me and said, "Are you okay? What is that?" Following those words, she was pointing to my heart scar. Then I realized I had never really been open to that many people about my heart. I was only open about it to those who needed to know about it. Then came Tuesdays. I strongly disliked middle school and Tuesday gym class. We had to run in a straight line and not pass each other for ten minutes. Guess who ended up being the slowest? If you guessed me, that is correct. Kids started talking, and rumors started spreading. But I believe word got out too that I did, in fact, have a heart condition, and I could not help it. Middle school is when I started learning to play the clarinet.

Middle school was also when I met my best friend. I do not remember much of my middle school life, but I do remember my principal, and every day, he would say, "Make it a great day or not; the choice is yours." How true is that?

## High School

Senior year, I felt like I had everything down. At the same time, I was so ready to get out of the school at the same exact time… My best friend in High School ended up graduating a year ahead of me. We did so much together. She moved to our little hometown and came to middle school with me, and that is where we met. We did so much together. She came over to my parents' place for slumber parties. She came over to my grandparents' place for my birthday party a few different times. We had every single kind of talk you could imagine. We talked about our future, weddings, kids, husbands, and what they were all going to be like. We talked about school, friends, family, yeah, just about anything and everything. After she graduated, we really did not talk for a couple of years. But many life things happen, and by God's grace, we were able to connect again. When we did start talking again, it was like we had never stopped talking. She is now engaged and will be married in 2020! I had one other girl that I would've considered a best friend. But senior year was a bit hard on our friendship. I never admitted to her that I wished she would not hide in the bathroom to talk to a guy. I often sat alone or felt alone once she left to go talk to him. She would do this every single day. The other people that sat around our table, I learned a bit later, really did not like me because I talked about God too much. I then chose to sit at another table where the friend that would run to the restroom would join me to eat quickly and then leave me alone for the rest of the lunch period. Sophomore and Senior years were the hardest for me. Those were the two years my heart acted crazy and did not love me at all.

In my sophomore year of High School Band camp, I was pre-approved to leave camp for a few hours and go back to camp when I was finished. My church at the time was going to put on a puppet show in the park the Sunday after I got home from band camp. Well, while I was practicing my puppet (I do not remember much but was told later), my heart raced 222 beats per minute, and I blacked out. The last thing I remember was trying to drink water. I remember the person in charge got us in the car and sped home. My home was with my parents. My parents rushed out the door, got me inside, and laid me down on my own bed. I was feeling fine, but I was in a panic that I had to get back to band camp; practice was over. My parents told me there was no way I was going back to band camp that night. I remember being mad and upset. I remember yelling about how my band teacher was going to be so mad that I did not report back to the band like I said I was going to. My parents woke me up early in the morning and took me to see my cardiologist. Her partner was in, but she was not in yet. My parents explained what had happened the night before, and they took me in immediately. I remember that I had not wanted to be there. I wanted to go back to band camp and be with my friends. We were coming home soon anyway.

"Do you feel better laying down or sitting up?" A nurse asked me.

"Laying down, I think, " I said.

The nurse helped me lay down, and I was out. I woke up in the Emergency Room at the same hospital. My dad was sitting next to me, and I gave him a quick help me look, and he walked over to me and started talking to me. I remember him starting to sing "Smile

Sweetheart Smile" by Frankie Yankovic. A short time later, a doctor came in and introduced himself to me. He told me I was going to meet "Old Sparky" that day but not to worry, he was going to put me to sleep. We had to go through some paperwork, and he told me there was going to be a small chance I would remember or feel the shock, but putting me to sleep would not make it feel as bad. I do not remember being shocked. I ended up somehow getting to the University of Michigan. I was there only a few days, but my doctor was trying to figure out what my heart was doing and what exactly was wrong with it. Then, it came time for an oblation. He said that if the oblation does not work, we would feel best if he put in an Implantable Cardiovascular Defibrillator or an ICD. When I woke up from this procedure, I looked over at my parents and said, "Well, do I have one, or did it work?" My dad shook his head and told me I have the ICD now. I reached over to my left side and felt my chest. Yep, I found it, and it felt different. There is no way to really describe what it feels like when you first wake up, and now you have a pacemaker and a defibrillator inside your chest. I was in my own room now at U of M, and I could not move for 6-8 hours. I had to stay on my back! I remember sleeping a lot or trying to sleep when I was not in a bunch of pain. My dad looked at me and said, "So are you going to name your device after your doctor who just spent eight hours on your heart, sitting and waiting and watching your heart? I never thought about naming my device. Who did that anyway? But after talking about it for a few minutes, I decided that I was going to name my device Little Dave Jr. A year and a few months passed. Then, my world went dark again.

Before my world went dark, I was at my local church in a class to become a member of the church. Honestly, I felt fine. I was a bit tired, but I had just finished running around with the kids. But I had food and water before class, so I felt fine. Out of nowhere, I ended up falling face-first in front of everybody in the class. The pastor called 911 one time, and people ran to the other room to get my parents. As I woke up, trying to make sense of what had just happened, there were paramedics all around me. I remember thinking, "Absolutely NOT! This is my Senior year of High School; my heart can not mess up or mess with me this year." But what came from my mouth? "Little Dave did it! Little Dave shocked me! Paramedics had no idea what I had met by that, so as to why I said that, it is what felt right, I guess. My Mom had to explain to the paramedics who were at the scene what Little Dave was. That was my first ambulance ride. I will say I do remember. I remember one of the paramedics would not shut up! I wanted him to just stop talking for a few minutes so that I could think about what in the world had just happened. But I also knew he was doing his job; he was talking to me, and I was replying. He wanted to keep me awake. He did not want me to pass out again. But of course, if I had, he and the team would be ready. I ended up talking his ear off and explaining my story of how I had gotten to this point in my life of having Little Dave Jr. We ended up going into a Bronson emergency room. Doctors again had a really hard time figuring out what it could have been. Finally, a representative came to my hospital bed to take readings off of Little Dave Jr. to see if I was right. To see if I was shocked for the first time in my Senior year of High school. After the company representative came and read what was on my device, it was confirmed I had been right. I was not shocked once, but twice in my church, in front of people.

I honestly do not remember much of what happened after that night. But at one point, I realized that I should be awake by now! I guess this next bit is something I have kept quiet for too long, but I remember fighting to wake up, feeling like I was trapped. I remember wanting to open my eyes, tap my fingers, move my toes, anything to alert someone I wanted to wake up or that I was waking up. Yet I heard not one person around me; it was dark, and I felt alone. It was like my soul was awake, but my body was not! I don't remember an out-of-body experience, though. I never saw myself laying where I was, wherever I was. After a few seconds of panic, I kind of remember trying to look up. I remember thinking, "I am scared, God, " my world went dark again.

I did wake up, and it did not feel like long after I was thinking about being scared. But where was I? What happened? I turned my head slowly, and I saw my dad. I tried to smile. Dad noticed and got up. I did not know where my mom came from, but all of a sudden, she was next to me, too. I tried smiling again. Mom turned away for a quick second, and I looked at my dad for reassurance. Mom was talking to me; I wanted to talk back. I looked up and noticed that she was looking down at me. She, too, was smiling. She started rubbing my forehead.

"How're you feeling, sweetie?" Mom asked.

Knowing sign language, I tried signing "OK," but it came out as a cough. I touched my throat. A nurse came in and gave me some Apple Juice. How in the world did she know I wanted that? Had I said I wanted it? I was grateful for it. I think mom asked the nurse for me, if it was alright that I could have some. Then, after I looked over at my parents and after some Apple Juice, I squeaked out a short, soft "Hi." I am not sure how long after that, I layed there. But what felt like only a few minutes, I had doctors and nurses talking around me. They were talking about moving me out of the ICU and into a room I could stay in till I was strong enough to go home. But they moved me soon after. I had the bed next to the window, too! Then I remembered something!

"Mom, I have to get out of here. I am in the puppet show on Sunday!"

"Honey, that was a few days ago. Today is Tuesday of the following week. You missed the performance; I am so sorry."

"Mom, I have another question."

"Okay dear, what is it?"

"Where am I"?

"University of Michigan, you are safe here."

After she told me where I was, I remember being confused again. How did I get here? I was at Bronson, not far from where I lived, and now, I am at the U of M, two hours away from the last place I remembered being.

The few days turned into a week, and the week turned into a week and a half, and it felt like I was never going to leave this hospital. Tests were not looking good at all. My heart function went way low and kind of quickly. I was going into heart failure! Maybe it is a good thing I do not remember the exact date it happened, but my doctor came in; he sat on the edge of my bed and smiled at me.

"How are you feeling today, Rach?"

I rolled my eyes when I heard him call me that. I honestly never liked anyone calling me Rach since the first time someone had tried.

"I am doing okay; I feel fine, really!"

"I know you do, but your heart is just not happy with you. How many times have I told you not to push yourself over what you know you can do? Anyway, there is something we need to talk about: you, me, and your mom and dad here."

What is happening to me! Why do I feel like I am fine, but my doctor says differently? I trust my doctor so much, but still.

My doctor pats my leg. "You're a fighter, I know. Your heart is trying to keep up with you and the active lifestyle that you want to live. But I want you to live more years, Rachel. I want you to keep growing and learning. But your heart function is way too low. Low enough, there is no easy way of saying it, but there is a high chance you will not leave this hospital until we get you on the heart transplant listings. You need a new heart to continue living your life to the fullest."

That, right there, was the absolute biggest pill to swallow at the age of 15! Did I sleep that night? Nope, not at all. I was in constant prayer. I was praying more and more because I was scared. The more I prayed about it, the more excited I was getting with the possibility of receiving a new heart. My prayer went from "God, why me?" to "God, your will be done." I was starting to look up at all the positive things that I could do with a new heart. I really started liking the idea of being able to play a sport; I was excited that I could learn something new. I was starting to pray God's Will be done and to keep showing me all of the positive stuff that I could learn and do with a new heart. I began to Thank God for the family and the person who would end up looking for his/her life to save mine. I started praying for the family. I wanted to live, but I knew someone else would have to die for me. During this stay in the hospital, I met a girl named Bridget. She had a pacemaker battery check and had to stay a couple of days (I can not remember why now, though). But we began to get close, I helped her adventure out of her room, she would come to mine and I could go to hers. We also had a craft room where we could go too. So we ventured out and went into the craft room as well. Bridget had a negative mindset, and I quickly learned I did not need that for myself in the hospital; I prayed about it. Within 24 hours after praying about it, she was well enough to go home. She would come and visit me (she did not live far away at the time) and bring me small gifts. We would hang out in one room, and our parents would be in another. With how low my heart function was, doctors seemed really impressed that I was even walking around, going to other rooms, making friends, and doing crafts. All these memories now feel like so long ago, but in reality, it is crazy to think about. It is currently 2019, so all of this took place eight years ago!? What is even more strange is that in two years, 2021, in October, it will be 10 years! I can not tell you the exact day or the time, but God pulled through again! He did another miracle.

## 2014

2014 started off a wonderful year! On May the 30th, 2014, I walked the stage and graduated! Doctors, my parents, and I, for a while, thought I would not make it to see graduation day! But I did!

## The Beat Goes On – 2019

The growing year for myself, 2019. So much had happened. God was working on my heart spiritually and at it again physically, too. This year, in particular, has been one of the hardest years that I can remember. You will never guess where I am at writing this section of this chapter. At the U of M, I have been admitted for the first time in six years. September 7th, 2019, my day started really well. I was at our Michigan Flywheelers tractor and engine show. I have gone to this event since I was three months old. There was nothing really out of the ordinary that day. My brother and I walked the majority of the flea market, spending money, laughing, and making a YouTube video to post later. Lunchtime comes and goes, and we decided that We should eat first before getting back out to the flea market to finish up what we had not seen yet. So we walked and got food. The food vendors are in the same row that we had camp set up, but I found it harder to get back to camp. I finally made it back to camp, and we showed Mom and Dad what all of us had gotten to eat. My siblings and friends had big plates of food; I had one small $4.00 taco and deep-fried Oreos. We all ate, But I felt extra tired and sore. I did not want to go walking anymore. My back, head, chest, I am not really sure how to describe it, but I was just tired and felt "done" for the day. I felt like I could use a long nap. So, I stayed behind. My brother was not happy with me but ended up going with his girlfriend and our sister instead. I stayed at camp. The parade was going to be at two. My siblings and their friends had gone to find a seat to watch the parade. The next big thing I remember is Dad is on this huge tractor in front of our camp, and he is pointing and waving at me to come with him. So I hopped on the tractor. I felt like I had power again! I had energy again; I was smiling, waving at people, and hanging on for dear life, trying to find a comfortable spot to sit or stand on the tractor. There was a person who was clearly not thinking at all who ended up walking right in front of our tractor. Dad saw them just in turn and hit the tractor emergency brake. The tractor halted to stop. I flung forward hard, but I was still holding onto the tractor. Dad kept asking if I was fine, and I replied out of breath that I was fine. After saying I was fine, I moved forward again a bit, and the conversation went something like…

Dad: What in the world was that? You okay?

Me: Well, actually….That really hurt.

Dad: What did…? (stops the tractor)

Me: I was shocked; I mean, I think I was. That really hurt.

Dad: Like from your device shocked?

Me: yeah, yes

Dad: (moves the tractor so it's now in line for the parade, but has me sit and leans on the steering wheel. Jumps from the tractor and gets on the phone)

My mom shows up, other family shows up to take over our tractor, and mom, dad, and I race the golf cart through people blowing the horn and yelling, Emergency!!!! We get to the car. Mom forgot her purse and car keys, so I stayed in the car. Mom stays with me, and Dad goes back through the crowd of people, back to the campsite to get Mom's purse. I spent four hours in Bronson ER. They sent me off to the U of M Emergency Department. I sign papers saying that I consent to my dad taking me instead of an ambulance or flight. Mom went to be with my siblings, and Dad drove me up to U of M. We both were not feeling the greatest. (Remember, I ate very little earlier) So we are in the Emergency Department at U of M, and I get a room. I spent 24-plus hours in the U of M Emergency Department because the hospital had run out of beds, where people were admitted. The emergency Department also ended up running out of rooms. So, I learned quickly to be thankful I could at least kind of sleep with a door shut for privacy. Just a quick side note: Bronson ER, I was in room 17, and in the Emergency Department, I was in room 27! At about 8:30 PM, I moved from the Emergency Department to my room, where I stayed for six days. There was a lot of just waiting. On

Monday, I had an Echocardiogram done. On my way to get it done, the lady who transported me was super friendly, chatty, and slow. The test took about an hour. Something was not right, so the person doing the test walked out and came back in. She tells me that they are going to inject this stuff into my IV, and what this stuff is supposed to do is make my heart more clear and easier to read. So as one other person is injecting this into my IV, the other person sees it go past my heart and takes pictures. These two women who did this did not really ask how I felt about it. My doctors had not ordered it, and I felt pressured into saying at least okay so that I could just get out of the Echocardiogram. I spent another 10 minutes waiting for someone to come get my bed so that I could go back to my room and cry everything out. A girl comes, and I tell her the info she needs, and she (It felt like) ran with my bed back to my room. I was very dizzy; the girl did not talk to me or try to make me even a little comfortable. I get back to my room, and I get up to walk around a bit. I go into the bathroom and just cry. I go back to my bed, and my tech person comes in and says, "Alright, are you okay? Can I hook you back up? I looked her straight in the face, and my mom said it for me.

"Something happened, and NO."

I shook my head No and said, "I want to see my nurse."

My nurse for the day was Mark, and he was the best nurse I had since being on the floor. I told him how I was feeling and let him hook me back up. He wrote down my feelings about what had just happened during my testing. He was not happy that I had to experience any of this. At the end of his shift, he came into my room and told me he had written up my case and what I had gone through that day.

The rest of my stay was a lot of just watching and waiting. I was there for six days. While there, they started me on Lasix. I was in the bathroom every half hour. That week, I lost 9 pounds of water weight from my body. The Echocardiogram showed that I had way too much water around my heart and in my body.

## One Year Later, December 13th 2019

Today is like a birthday (I'm officially 24.5 today, if that counts) to me. (It's not why I'm celebrating, though)You have a special day in mind, and when it finally becomes the first of that month, it feels like it drags until the day is actually here! Then it's hard to believe that the day, a special day, has finally come. Then you ask yourself, when the day is here, what am I going to do with my day? I wish I had a picture of me a year ago today... A year ago today, I left what was comfortable to me. What was comfortable to me, not one person should be comfortable with ever! I left a boy I had been dating one day shy of 4.5 years. Today, I celebrate being single and free! Today, I celebrate that I have a wonderful new home church to grow with; I have friends, both new and "old." Everyone and everything I really did love. I lost the day I said yes to him, but the day I said NO MORE and YES to JESUS, I got everything and much more back. For the first time in 5 years, I put on my promise ring from Papa God/Dad, and it still fits! Their love for me never shrunk. They just kept loving me and waited till I came home. It feels so good to feel connected again to the right people and to King Papa God!

These are my top three life verses!

And the God of all grace, who called you to his eternal glory in Christ, after you have suffered a little while, will himself restore you and make you strong, firm, and steadfast. 1 Peter 5:10.

Though you have made me see troubles, many and bitter, you will restore my life again. From the Depths of the earth, you will increase my honor and comfort me once more! Psalms 71:20-21.

So do not fear, for I am with you; do not be dismayed, for I am your God. I will strengthen you and help you; I will uphold you with my righteous right hand. Isaiah 41:10.

A year ago today, I prayed for a life verse, for God to show me something. I have learned so much in a year; it's hard to believe, but I lived it, and God did it!

Side note: the earrings pictured are the first ones I bought because I chose them and did not ask for approval from anyone. Today, I wear them to remind myself I don't need man's approval; I've got God's. I listen to God.

## 2020 is going to be another Learning year? I think so!

Every new year should be a learning year. A person should not stop learning. A person should never have the attitude like they know everything because, truth be told, only God knows everything and everything. You can not hide anything from God. Last year, 2019, I thought was going to be a hard year, but I have learned this. Indeed, it was a hard year, but there are different kinds of hard years a person may go through. 2019 - I was single for the first time in four and a half years and learned who I wanted to be and what I wanted to do. And in 2019, my family had many deaths of friends. 2020, though, is going to be my heart, learning how to rest and trusting God in a new way.

# Happy New Year!

## 2020 - Being Remade

I am beyond excited that I am in my 20s in the new 20's! This is absolutely crazy awesome that we are already in a new decade. I am excited to see what this decade has in store for me. I know my Open Heart surgery is coming up soon; it may be closer than we think! I finally found a dentist who will take me in as a patient and is not afraid to help me just because I have a lot going on, both in my mouth and my heart.

## Losing my Job, Not my Identity

My Identity is in Christ. Who am I? I am a woman of God, God's child. I am a sister in Christ/ This is who I am, and I am very proud of who I am. This is something God keeps reminding me on a daily basis now. I lost my job Wednesday, January 15th, 2020. According to the policy, it is three write-ups, and you're out. But also, according to the write-ups, I was supposed to sign them. I never did because I had no idea I even had them. It also talks about talking to an admin, and they signed it after I was too. That never did happen. One admin just signed it and wrote instructions above where I was to sign, so there would not even be room for me to sign if I were to sign them. Then also two in one day? Is that even legal? So I went on Wednesday, and I feel like that should have been my warning day, especially because two were from the only other day that I worked.

## February 2020 - God is my love story

We are three days into February. I have not heard from the ex. Good. At this point, I wish we could just live our own lives that God has for each of us. We are on good terms now, as far as I know. Thank you, Papa God, for that. Now, to move on with life.

2020 already had its own challenges in my life. I am working on just telling you the truth, but I worked really hard to keep it all positive. But life has been hard. Becoming an adult has been hard. As mentioned already, losing my job was really hard; the kids that I worked with, my friends I was starting to make, all of a sudden, I was not there, week after week. Others have left since I had been let go. But now February is here; I just paid my phone bill, and I am under fifty dollars in my savings account. I do not even have enough to pay for next month's phone bill! I have a job interview tomorrow, and I am super excited about this. Today, I also got a call to set up a phone interview somewhere else. So, working on staying positive; my resume is getting out there, and now I am praying that the right people are seeing it!

## March 2020 - Open Heart Surgery number two

### Monday, March 2nd, 2020

I walked into the University of Michigan hospital, knowing I would be staying awhile. I was on floor seven, and every single nurse I had must have been great because I do not remember having a bad one my first week in the hospital. Thursday, March 5th, I had all four of my Wisdom teeth pulled in the Dentistry part of U of M. I needed this done to be okayed for my open heart surgery. I was in there for about an hour and a half. I had one tooth that the dentist could not get out and was trying to get a surgeon to help her get it out, but then we turned on Matthew West's music, and as I was worshiping in my head, that tooth just came out. She got it without the surgeon. My roommate was super awesome and very encouraging. I learned a little later that she loves Jesus just like I do.

**Monday, March 9th, 2020**

I cleaned up at four in the morning and was wheeled down to surgery preparation. I refused a pregnancy test because I did not have to use the bathroom, and I was also one hundred percent sure I was not. They had me wash my mouth out with something that almost made me sick right before surgery. After all, I haven't eaten anything since before midnight. I got back into the preparation bed, and a person who does IVs came in and put one in my arm. I honestly can't remember what arm, though. As I am being prepped for surgery, I now have Josh's sweatshirt over me to help me keep warm, and I also felt like I was being comforted with it on top of me as well. I knew there was a small chance of waking up and seeing Josh, and he knew that too, but I told him I would feel when he was there and I would know. He walked in, and I opened my eyes. I don't remember actually seeing him, but I woke up and could tell he was standing next to me. I remember lifting up my arm, trying to touch his face; he bent low (probably to tell me to lay back down or that I was okay), and then I touched his face; I felt his facial hair and knew he was there. I could picture him now standing there. I laid back down, my breathing tube came out, and I crocked a "Hi baby!"

The short time that Josh and I were together, would you believe I had yet another one of my episodes? We were out together with family, listening to Richards' Magic Accordion live! We were on the dance floor dancing, and I was teaching him how to polka dance when everything felt right, and then it wasn't. I got really dizzy, had a headache, my vision started narrowing in, and I started slowing down. But I didn't fall? I found out a little bit later that I was, in fact, going to fall, but Josh had caught me in my fall, and my family helped me get to the chair I was in. Now I'm in a chair, and I'm trying to breathe. Music has stopped, and I notice people leaving. Then I scream a murderous scream! My device shocked me. Everyone around me knew it, too. I didn't have to say anything. Sitting in the chair it was hard to stay sitting up. I wanted to lie down and sleep.

I found myself saying, "Make it stop"!

While sitting down trying to breathe, my ICD had shocked me, not once but four times that night. (That's the most my ICD had ever shocked me at one time) So my parents and Josh got me into our truck and took me straight to U of M this time. The ride there was a blur. I laid on Josh while my dad and him were talking to me trying to keep me awake. I remember feeling annoyed because I knew they didn't want me to pass out, but I was tired. All I remember upon arrival was that it was about 10:30-11:15 PM when we got to the Emergency Department, and I had a room pretty quickly. I knew this would be another hospital stay, and I was right. They found me a room fairly quickly. By the time I was in the system, I thought I could sleep; they were waking me up for 6 AM blood draws and vitals even though I had just had them. This particular stay, I don't remember how long, but doctors were concerned if I needed a shock again; with what I had, it was not strong enough to bring me back like it had done the night before after four shocks. My doctor ended up adding a lead around my heart. This gave me three leads now instead of two. One being added was in hopes of making the delivery shock stronger, so I would only need one shock if I ever needed another shock.

## Intensive Care Unit - Monday, March 16th

I was still in the Intensive Care Unit (ICU).

I was really ready to get out of there. You see, my ICU experience was not the greatest. I had several very rude nurses. I hate taking Potassium now. I had several nurses try and do the powder stuff and have me drink it, but every time I did, I would throw up everything. This happened four times! One nurse, in particular, made me try the powder stuff again, saying most people like it this way instead; she stood there in front of me after telling her I would though up again if I did this, and she told me to drink it, chug it and I would not feel a thing, she promised nothing would happen. After gulping three or so, I put a blanket over me, and I threw up. Then she seemed mad at me and treated me differently because now she had to clean me up. Her voice was louder when she talked to me, and she acted like she did not like me or could not handle being around me. They thought I was still under anesthesia, and that is why I refused the powder. By day six or seven after surgery, I had nurses comparing me to "normal people." They would say things like, "Normally, people, after surgery on day three, have a bowel movement, and you still have not."

They would try so hard to give me the medication that they stick up my butt to help me have a bowel movement. I kept taking a pill that would soften the bowel movements, but not nothing was coming. I finally had one, and a nurse told me that it was too small, and she ordered the pill that went up my butt. This may be too much info, but I took it. But nothing happened in the ICU. They were all small and not "big enough." I was tired of being compared to "normal people." Then came the Virus outbreak and fear. So, while I was still in ICU, they told everyone to go home, and that was not a patient. This meant that both of my parents had to leave me! They had been in my room with me, and now, in the blink of an eye, I was fighting for myself, trying to understand everything that was happening to me. Mom called my cardiologist nurse, who got really upset. My mom and dad were home after I had the major invasive surgery. They made the announcement at 9:45, and everyone had to be out by 10:00 in the morning. My mom called my cardiologist's nurse, who had to pull a few strings here and there and finally, a parent could come back. But by then, I had left the ICU. The more I started to understand what was happening around me.

I do not remember the exact day, but it was after they told me I would be going to a new floor and to a new room. A nurse came in and took everything I knew in the ICU was taken away from me. No warning. They told me I was going to a new room. I was excited at first; they found a bed for me, but then, who took my bed? I was being moved, yes, to another ICU room. I was so disappointed and hurt. Not one person came in and explained why. That is, until the day I was actually leaving the ICU, a male nurse who was a charge nurse, told me it was because they needed my room for an emergency ICU virus patient. I gave him my thoughts on it, how I was moved, and no one till now came to talk to me about why I was being moved. Want to know why I was moved? They needed my room for a serious case of the virus if one were to come into the ICU.

## There is Good in the Dark

I met a Tec named Shelly. She was fantastic! She was the light in this dark place. She had seen me right after surgery to see me getting up and walking the ICU floor. I can guarantee you that when you're struggling, she will try and make your day better. When Josh called, she heard his ringtone and then asked me what type of music I was into. I told her about several Christian songwriters, and she knew most of my favorites. In fact, she had a list of Christian songs on her phone to share with me. We would play one from the list and sing it out loud together. The team knew I really liked Shelly. I asked for a musical therapy person to come in to help, and they sent Shelly in. so then we would turn up the music again and worship together in the ICU.

Not every nurse was bad. There was one nurse who stuck out to me because she spoke kindly to me, was helpful, tried to understand me, and helped me throughout her day shift. She helped me want to get out of bed, get up, stretch, and walk around the ICU floor. Her name was Umeko! She was awesome! If I had two awards to give out, they would go to Shelly and Umeko!

## Papa God in the ICU

I was falling asleep in my chair. But I felt like a door opened behind me. (There was no door behind me) Then something walked in, rubbed my shoulders, touched my arms, and kissed me on the forehead. Then I felt something whisper, "It is all going to be alright; I've got you, you're safe!" I woke up and asked my mom if she felt that. She said, "Rosalie, felt what? That is when I realized it was the Holy Spirit. I had literally heard and felt the Holy Spirit in a new way. It was at first kind of scary, but as I realized what was happening, I wanted to continue to feel it.

## Moving on up, New Floor

I was finally moved up to floor four. This room God was in, and I could feel it. He really did have me. I was getting frustrated because I knew I had to go to floor four before I could go home, but I kept praying for specifics. I wanted Bed two, and I wanted to be with a roommate who knew Jesus and loved Jesus. Was that way too much to ask for? Finally, in frustration, I prayed:

"God, at this point, I don't care what bed I get. It would be nice to have a Christian woman as a roommate, but if I am supposed to witness to someone then put us together, I am just tired of feeling healthy and still in the ICU. I just want to go home!" I love you, and I know you can get me out of here, please Papa, help me"!

Within an hour, my cardiologist comes into my ICU room to say hello, listens to my heart, tells me how great it sounds, listens to my breathing, and then tells me, "I think you're moving on up; they got a bed for you upstairs!"

I was so excited I started to cry happy tears. He shook my hand and smiled at me.

Shelly and my nurse that day ended up taking me to my room. 125-2. Prayers were answered. I had bed two, so I had the window side. My roommate, we will call her Molly, looked to be close to eighty years old. Her surgery was going to be that Thursday. So I had Tuesday and all day Wednesday to talk to her and get to know her. A physical therapist came in and showed Molly some exercises she was going to have to do after her surgery. The physical therapist started showing her how to march so she could start moving her legs a little bit. That is when Molly burst into the song, "I may never march in the infantry, ride in the cavalry, shoot the artillery, but I am in the Lord's Army"!

That is when I knew God had answered yet another prayer. My roommate loved Jesus. That same night, I got up to my new room. Doctors wanted a chest x-ray. So I was wheeled away for a chest x-ray, and Molly spoke up and said:

"You're not taking that sweet girl away already, are you?

My nurse replied, "She has a small test, and then she will be back."

Miss Molly just laid back and smiled.

"Okay" was all she said.

I also learned that she was a Sunday school teacher a long time ago. There was a pastor at U of M (recently retired) that she had in her Sunday School class.

One night, a food service worker said

"Have a good night, ladies. Goodnight.

She then started singing "Goodnight Irene."

I know of this song because my dad plays it on his accordion.

The night of Molly's heart surgery, I had a very hard time sleeping. I was physically alone. Her husband came in about 3:30 that morning, and he was very chirpy for being awake so early in the morning. Yes, he woke me up, but I was honestly okay with him waking me up. I sat up in bed, shed a few tears, and prayed. I literally had nothing else to do but sleep, and that was almost going to be impossible by now. I was so worried for Miss Molly. I asked Papa God to help me sleep because I knew that I needed to try and sleep. The next twenty-four hours, God knew how much I was worrying about this beautiful human, and honestly, I do not think I have prayed that much in a full twenty-four-hour period for one specific person. My heart wanted to know how Molly was doing. I believe that God (knowing all) saw my heart, wanting to know how she was doing. A day or two later, my nurse came in, smiled at me, and told me I was getting a new roommate. That is when I saw Molly's wheel around into our room! I burst into pure joy and tears! She made it. She was going to be okay! The physical therapist came in to work with her and tried having her move her feet; she sang, "I may never March…"

Now, my mom was with me; she asked me what was wrong. I told her that it was Molly; she was the one who did all the singing all week and how that had kept my spirits up. Of all the rooms at U of M, They chose to put her with me, or they thought they could try and put her with me. Only God can give you your old roommate your new roommate again!

# COVID-19

I honestly tried to avoid the above topic. But I can't. The world is changing so much, and so are we. The world is hurting, and so are we. I personally have been in a lock-up situation since March second of twenty-twenty. So, a week before my Open Heart Surgery. But just another way God is good and took care of me. I got my surgery the week before quarantine and before everything was going to be on lockdown. Doctors and Nurses started kicking people out who were visitors, and others were cancelling surgeries.

## Two months post Open Heart Surgery.

Many things have changed just in the two months since my Open Heart Surgery. Life is still not normal. The state of Indiana is slowly getting out of being quarantined now. Michigan is still quarantined till the 28th of May as of right now. I am praying so hard that life starts to get back to a new normal. Staying inside has been so hard. Then I can start getting myself out there and actually dating again. So I am sad to say Josh and I did not last very long. I liked him, but we moved way too fast. On our first date, we made it official only after knowing each other for maybe a week. I want to get to know someone as a friend first before we move on; I am afraid of getting attached too soon and something happening. One day, I am going to trust a man wholeheartedly. He knows my story and accepts me for who I am.

## Five months post Open Heart Surgery

Life has been busy! 2020 has been a hugely challenging year. I can not believe it is already August! From a medical point of view, I am stable. I am meeting my new electrophysiologist this month, and we are discussing a new upgraded pacemaker/Defibrillator. This device is going to be bigger with more battery life since I am being paced close to 70 percent of the time.

Family-wise, we are all hanging in there. This sounds scary, but I am actually engaged now. Michigan came out of quarantine on May 22$^{nd}$, 2020. That was when the gatherings could start up again slowly anyway. So, on May 22$^{nd}$, I met a man I had been talking to for a few weeks over video. We have been inseparable since. So he asked me to be his wife! Yes, you read that correctly. I am going to be a wife. I am engaged! The end of this month I am going Wedding Dress shopping. COVID-19 still thinks it is under control; I can only take two other people with me to the dress shop. I am taking my grandma Nancy and my mom. Grandma never got the chance with my mom to go dress shopping, and my mom never got to try on dresses, So I want to make them feel special too and make them feel like they are a part of my decisions for the wedding.

Speaking of my Grandma, Her sister is not doing very well right now. The family has decided to call in hospice, and my aunt has quit dialysis. She has talked about how she is ready to go be with her mom and dad and her younger sister. (Who also died of heart complications at a young age) How she is excited to meet Jesus and see his face. She wants to be buried at her father's feet. This has been one crazy year!

## Eight Months Post Open Heart Surgery

It is the end of November. In just a few weeks, I will be nine months from my Open Heart Surgery. My story continues, though. I am still engaged! He learns more about my heart and still wants me. This is a wonderful sign. I love this man more than he will ever know. He has taught me what true love feels like. How deep our souls are and how connected we are. He has really connected with my family, and even though my siblings were hesitant at first, they are making a wonderful effort to get to know the man that I love. I love watching my brother and his bond the most.

My sister is now engaged. We are getting married five months apart. We are in May of 2021, and they are in October of 2021.

As far as my grandma's sister/my great aunt, she has passed. She is with Jesus now. I got to call her and tell her all about my husband-to-be, our plans, how I have my dress, veil, flowers and my bridal party! She told me to have a great life, and then we hung up. That was super hard.

December is going to be interesting this year. I can't wait to see what God is going to do. December 7th, my heart surgeon is going to put new wires around my heart in hopes that this will have my heart beat together instead of beating separately. Then, on December 9th, exactly nine months post my open heart surgery, I got a new device with more battery that is made to pace my heart for longer amounts of time and last a really long time.

As of COVID-19, Life is happening. Some people think it is a big old joke; others are so scared about it that they are still staying home and letting fear overtake them. We need to live our lives. I can't stay home and do nothing. I am at work, the store, or home. Yes, I am going back to church too. But our church is being very careful, and we are six feet apart; we are wearing our masks, and I, with my condition, only a selected few get to hug me and touch me. The cases were going down or being stable, but they are currently going back up again, which means I can not have a visitor with me at all at the hospital when I have my two surgeries.

## Ten Month Update

I feel like my story just keeps on going. This is a very good thing, though. It is now January of 2021! (I worked on drafts of this book way too long, haha, still proud of it.)

In my eight-month post, I mentioned two surgeries. Well, I only had one. But there is a positive to this. There is a new heart device that is being studied. My heart meets all of the requirements for this new trial device. The first surgery I was going to have was going to do what this trial device is made to do. I have missed working in a family-owned restaurant since I had it back in 2018. That is when I learned I really do love it, but it depends on the people around you. I start this job next week. I was let go six days later after my surgery, but five days later, it was bleeding everywhere, and I ended up back in the hospital for another six days. Since I have a pre-existing condition, I am next in line to get the COVID-19 vaccination. My cardiologist believes it is safe and is telling me I should get it.

My grandma is not doing well, and the family is having a hard time. I spent about twelve weeks with her as her caregiver before we decided to put her in a home last year. So maybe that was my grieving time, and now I am waiting for her to physically leave the earth before I show any more emotion. She ended up in the hospital, and the doctor suggested bringing her in hospice. If she stays on earth just this year (2021), it will be a miracle.

## God Provides

I thought I would take a few minutes to talk about how else God has provided for us. My father was in a motorcycle accident at the end of last year. My father ended up "walking" out of the emergency room the same day with only a broken leg. The broken leg was honestly from the deer who decided to commit suicide that day. Well, his short-term disability had stopped, and we had a month of stuff that we needed but almost no money for the month. Someone donated to the church a money gift card for food, and our church was praying for who to give it to. The church, not knowing much of what we had been through, offered us a gift card that paid for all of the food for the month of February.

## One Year Post Open Heart Surgery

I have made it a full year and two days past my open-heart surgery date. March 9th, 2021, was actually a very good day. I got up about 6:30 in the morning and went to work! I am finally working full time now, again! I have not worked full-time in about a year. I am now a preschool teacher working in a school, in the school system. I have my own classroom full of students who look forward to coming to school to see what new song, project, or idea I have. As of the month of March, Austin and I have 72 days left until we become one. Being "in COVID times," we have our days where it is so wonderful while other days we struggle. With 72 days left for our wedding, all that we have left are guys' rentals, My dress alterations, and Decorations. My sister and I, along with my Godmother, are going to hand-make our decorations.

## Pray about it and then Listen

This is hard to do. It is easier said than done, and I completely understand. But God continues to provide if you listen and obey. Austin and I had looked at a small apartment in GR. But I had a gut feeling, "This is nice, but not ours." At this time, I was still unemployed. I was looking at jobs, but I could not find one that I would enjoy. I did not want to pick up a job that I would not enjoy. I started praying about living in GR and that I found a job that God would allow me to have and that my future husband was excited for me to have. Then, an email came. I wanted to apply but knew we were still going to move to GR, and if I got this dream job of mine, how was I going to get to work with one car? So, I missed the deadline. However, I applied for another position at a school, and honestly, I ignored them for about three weeks because we were still looking for jobs in GR for me, and KZOO was just too far away. But then, the school called me and got a hold of me. They were looking for a full-time person. So I talked to the person, I showed what I knew, and within a few hours, I knew this was where I belonged. Then, after talking about it and actually accepting the job, I got a call from the apartment place, and we got approved for our first apartment! When you listen, God will guide you. Please just ask and listen.

## Now, in my heart world

I am so blessed to have found a man who loves every single bit of me. I am so happy we got married on our one-year anniversary. Why? My heart is currently not doing well at all. Doctors have been talking about open heart surgery number three, and if that were not to do well, I would be ready to be listed for a heart transplant. So I had to go through numerous tests so that if I needed to be on the heart transplant list, they could just put me on. On August 4th of twenty twenty-one, I found out that they could not save the heart that I currently have. My heart function is way too low, and my heart from my previous heart surgery has healed to my chest bone, so opening my chest for heart surgery number three is just too dangerous. As of August 14, I need two more tests for doctors to have to review my case and put me on the heart transplant list. There are six stages of needing a new heart. I am on stage four because I was born with a weak, sick heart. When I get listed, the earliest I could get a heart is anywhere from three to six months, but everybody's journey is different when waiting for a heart.

## Steps to a new heart

On August 16th, 2021, I went and saw the hospital's dentist. Having a weak heart, I need to take amoxicillin before any kind of dental procedure, big and small alike. This is nothing new; I have always had to take medication before dental procedures because of my heart. So, what did I find out today? I need three more teeth pulled, possibly four; a few cavities need to be filled, and maybe a root canal; if one can be saved, she will. My dentist is a female who is around my age, I think. She seemed to calm me down. Austin was able to come back and be in the room with me. Going through all this stuff and having someone come back with me is a blessing. It keeps my anxiety down by more than half. I am also very blessed to have a husband to remind me in my moments of freaking out that God is in control and God knows what we can and can not handle.

September 7th, 2021. Not many know now, but soon, my readers, many will know. This is almost a raw moment of my feelings going through what I am. Let's consider this like a journal entry, except now it is public. I now have a Cyst. I have had it for some time. Just got it checked, but I am still worried. Bleeding more than normal and in so much pain that it hurts more, do I dare say more than a lot of the heart stuff I have been through? Living paycheck to paycheck is hard, and going to bed to cry and ask God why? I get it. I get you and understand you. Trying to learn to budget, but then it feels like you're out of money even sooner. Yep I know. I understand. Trying to keep your mind off food and trying to stay busy to push the hurt down, I sadly do not like to admit, but I get that too. When you cry and ask family for help, but they just turn their back, ohh, dear reader, I understand that too. But you are here for a reason; you picked this book for a reason. We may have been through a lot, but can I remind you and myself of one thing? God is in control, and he knows what he is doing. Know that there are people out there who understand because they have been there. These people are hard to find, but when you do, it feels amazing. We may be struggling in this life, but in all honesty, There is no one I would rather struggle with than the person I love the most. My husband and our fur child, who I want to swear, know more than we may think she does.

## Michigan vs. State

### October 30th 2021

This is now a day that is hard for me to process, and writing it out here helps. The University of Michigan was winning, but Michigan State made a comeback and ended up winning. Austin and I ordered delivery and decided to watch some TV. I had not felt great for about a week and a half, and I ended up passing out, and Boaz (my device) shocked me twice. Austin called 911 as I was sitting up and could hear him. I told him, too. After a night in one Emergency room, I dismissed myself and went up to U of M. I called ahead of time so U of M was ready for me. I became an inpatient that night. After many tests, doctors discovered my thyroid was way hyperactive, and I have a cyst! So, while figuring out heart stuff, they also tried to do other things that were not heart-related. The teams had talked about removing it during this stay. But the risks were just too high. Let's get it under control with medications if possible.

With God, ALL things are possible!

Well, that stay was twenty-one days! I came home the day before Austin, and I could celebrate six months of being married. So November twenty-first.

# Happy New Year!

This health stuff would not give me the slightest break. New year hit, and on day two, I was at U of M for follow-up checkups.

## March 2022

We are still waiting. Soon, this will be a full year of just talking about transplants. I am a bit annoyed as well about it. But let's just keep moving forward!

God has his own timing.

I am now down half of what I was on for steroids and found out I am allergic to one they originally had me on. I started getting red spots from the bottom of my legs, and each week, I noticed more. This was after they tried increasing it. I was fine till then. We are currently stuck again, not knowing things because the thyroid doctors say it is too high of a risk till after I get a new heart, but the transplant team, I think, wanted my thyroid removed first. This is how I personally understood it. So, all eight of my teams are coming back together to discuss what to do next. March 9th, 2022, will be two years already with Ruth. (My mechanical heart valve)

## April 2022

### The C word…

After two and a half years of being super careful, it hit me. On April 21st, 2022, I was diagnosed with Covid 19! I went through several emotions all at once. My test was supposed to take twenty-four to forty-eight hours for results. Well, I got mine in forty-five minutes from the swab. My first emotion was excitement. We had answers to why my energy kept going down, and my weight was going up. Austin could stay home to help me, and I could stop hearing, "It's all in your head."

That quickly changed to me being in shock. Covid did it. I found myself unprepared just once, and boom. After thinking about this, I cried. While crying, fear swept in. When Covid first started and was new, I got it in my head that if I ever got this, that was the end of my life.

Yes I was vaccinated. No, I did not do a booster because of all the heart side effects, and my team of doctors were unsure if I needed the shock if it would work or not.

So here we are, my first full day living with heart failure and Covid. My doctors and I made a decision the day I was diagnosed with it to try a medication ...but it had to be authorized. I had to meet certain criteria to get this medication. My pre-existing heart problems, along with my heart now failing, are what pushed me over enough to qualify. This medication somehow blocks the virus from spreading and creating. So, after only two doses of this, I got some things done.

- Took a shower

- Changed my clothes

- Did 95 percent of my dishes

If you have ever had Covid, you know how hard it can be just to get up and out of bed.

Everybody is different, so what were my symptoms?

- Light headed

- No energy

- Headache a lot of time

- Nausea

- Vomiting

- Loss of smell

- Loss of taste

- Cough

- Muscle aches. (Hands and hips)

- Shortness of breath during small activities. IE: climbing stairs.

I am trying so hard to find the mini miracles through this experience. God provides before you can even think about what you need. I'm so used to doing things myself because of heart failure. I want to push myself and do things. I want to be able to keep going like I used to, but I can not. It is hard admitting I need help, want help, or accept help. My friends on Facebook have no idea I have Covid. My family does, but I have asked them not to post. So instead, I'll post something like, "Life update: Not ready to say much. But I was going to U of M today. I've been so sick these past few days that my teams are in contact with me pretty much daily right now, but I canceled the appointment I had for today. That was a choice we made together with my transplant nurse and I, along with starting a new medication. I have a list of foods that do not stay down and a list of foods I can sort of tolerate or tolerate. I'm so glad I am not alone and have Austin and Riley, who right now are the only two who can be with me."

You quickly learn who cares, who loves you, and truly wants what is best for you. So there was a lady from the church where we got married who kept on commenting, telling me she'd been praying for me and would not stop. So I messaged her and told her that I have Covid. She made us dinner, got a few groceries for us, and left them at our doorstep. Giving in and saying Yes to dinner somehow relaxed me enough to go back to sleep. Austin baked it for us, and when it was done, we spent time watching a movie and eating.

## May of 2022

May has come quickly. May is here and soon will be gone. I will be 27 a month from today. As of today, all of us kids are basically on our own. Scary thought, that is, right? Austin and I are celebrating two years together, one year married in just nine more days. So much has happened in this book, just a few short chapters again, and we are in the new year! Hahaha, what! I learned something today, and I was slightly ticked off by it. I guess when I was told I was still in the hospital, all medicated up, it did not register all the way. But anyway, I had a doctor call me and tell me it was time for my annual checkup tests for the year. So all of those tests that I did a year ago for transplant I have to do again.

Austin and I have one month and twenty days till our next move. I'm not really looking forward to it too much. I am more scared of this move than when we moved out of my parents' place.

I got accepted into another small group, this time women. I know who the group leader is, and we have known each other for a long time now. Well, it feels like it's been a long time, but we honestly have been friends for three or four years now. I hope I will get along with everyone in that group. My mom says I will because she is in the group as well. So this is something I am looking forward to when we do move. There was also a church in town that did not hesitate to help us out with rent. So Austin and I are going to go visit them sometime this May. I want to give the pastor and the church a Thank you card for helping us out. Some of them know me and my story, but most just know I need a new heart and have been praying for me.

## July 11th - A big day SURPRISE

I was sitting in my room, and a doctor came in my room and said we accepted a heart for you. Honestly, I do not remember much after that. I woke up three weeks later. People often ask me how much I actually remember. But what I experienced was absolutely amazing. It felt like my brain was awake, and I saw people and different places.

John 14:2-3: In my Father's house, there are many mansions: if it were not so, I would have told you. I am going to prepare a place for you. And if I go and prepare a place for you, I will come again and receive you unto myself; that where I am there you maybe also.

I want to share where I went in an earthly time of three weeks but what felt like minutes to me before waking up.

Room 1: I was in a living room, with monitors. I knew of children in the room; however, I did not see any of them. I was laying down looking up at a TV, and the show seemed to be talking to the kids when, all of a sudden, there was a booming sound. Toys went everywhere. The teacher I loved being I wanted the kids to listen to me. I thought that I was in charge. Then, what seemed to be a toddler came in the doorway and told me, "Mom won't be mad." Then I shut my eyes to breathe and walked into room 2, The kitchen.

Room 2: The Kitchen. I was not here very long. I was laying down on a counter, and the father of the house was trying to put in a feeding tube by himself. I looked into the dining room, and I saw Pizza and coke. The father of the house asked if I would like to stay and eat with them, but first, we had to get that feeding tube in my nose. I saw what looked like a boy looking out the kitchen window, waiting for something or someone. There also seemed to be a wife figure who said

"You can stay awhile here; we have plenty."

Room 3: Bathroom: This was a beautiful room. Figure eight bath tub. It was black and white. There were Red flower petals around, and the water was running. There were candles lit also. I wanted to get in the tub and clean myself. I wanted to clean myself for something big. But then I heard a voice trying to calm me and telling me to lay back down.

"Child, it is not your time yet. Lay back down and relax."

In John, Chapter thirteen, The night before Jesus is to die on the cross, He gives his last meal to his disciples. Jesus took off his outer layer of clothes and put a towel around his waist, went around the table and washed his disciples' feet. When he got to Peter, a conversation between Jesus and Peter starts.

Verse 6: When Jesus came to Simon Peter, Peter said to him,

"Lord, are you going to wash my feet?"

Verse 7: Jesus replied, "You do not understand now what I am doing, But someday you will.

Verse 8: "No," Peter protested, "you will never ever wash my feet!"

Also, in verse eight, Jesus replies, "Unless I wash, you won't belong to me.

The conversation continues, and Peter wants Jesus to wash his entire body then.

Jesus replies in verse ten. Verse ten states that Jesus replied, "A person who has bathed all over does not need to wash, except for the feet to be entirely clean and you disciples are clean, but not all of you." Jesus knew who would hurt him and betray him. It was one of his own, Judas. The night Jesus was to die, Judas would bring the soldiers to him and kiss him on the cheek to show the soldiers who to arrest and kill.

Room 3: The porch. This room was harder to be in. I saw what looked like a Kitchen, and people were eating brunch, having contests, and getting special chairs. From where I was laying down, I could see what seemed to be about an eight to ten feet tall serving container. This container was full of orange Juice. I heard people talking about me.

"Mom, can we go give some to Rachel"?

"She is in the other room sleeping right now."

I tried screaming. I was awake and wanted some orange juice. Then a nurse-like figure came in, and when I asked if I could get up and join my family, she told me no, I needed to lay down. I could see my dad and brother in the other room, not sure where my mom and sister were. But on this porch, I laid down and looked the other way, and I saw now it was dark, and maybe they went home? I felt like I was wide awake in this porch bed; the couch, ceiling and mini fireplace all looked like they had wood on them for decoration or it was built like a log cabin. There was another room that looked and even smelled like a log cabin.

Leviticus 40 verses 40-41, the message bible in says, "On the first day, pick the best fruit from the best trees; take fronds of palm trees and branches of leafy trees and from willows by the brook and celebrate in the presence of your God for seven days. (41) Yes, for seven full days, celebrate it as a festival to God. Every year from now on, celebrate it in the seventh month.

ote: I find this amazing because my surgery was on the eleventh day of the seventh month of two thousand and twenty-two. Also, I was looking and praying for God to show me a verse to share for as many rooms as I could, and when my mom Googled Orange Juice, the above verses showed up first.

Room 4: The extra bedroom/living room. I felt like I was in someone's extra bed. A couch that turned into a bed. This room had a TV, pictures on the walls. On the shelves, there was another huge serving container, not as big as the first, but this time it had water. I started to feel thirsty now, seeing all these drinks in these different rooms. So a nice lady comes out, we get talking, I try and sit up to prove I can so that I could eat since it had been days that I have not had anything to eat or drink for awhile now. The nice lady said no, I could not have any. Just like everybody else around here is telling me. No. That is all I get nowadays, No. I thought to myself.

Room 5: This was the scariest of all of them. On the outside, it looked like a cute little barber shop. Inside, it was dark, and the basement was cold. The chairs looked like dentist chairs with straps.

These straps would hold down the victim so that the people in charge could do what they needed to do. A place I would never want to go back. The walls had moving objects on them. It looked like humans were also trying to escape but could not. The people or things in charge were trying to give me tattoos and a clean, old brushing on my teeth. I remember trying to scream for help. I finally had gotten a few words out.

"I have to be at grandma's house by a time." I finally said quietly.

"No one cares and is not looking for you; you might as well sit up and join us."

I remember fighting not to sit up this time but also trying to see if anyone was coming around the corner to rescue me from where I was. This was the first time I had not heard the father-like voice trying to calm me. I felt alone and scared. I kept hoping that my grandma was going to come look for me, and it was getting late, so the more I began to freak out and get scared.

## Coming back to Earth

The last room was a quicker visit; I was beginning to see reality now. I was back in a hospital room, on a bed, and I saw my dad smiling my way. I heard mom's voice and felt Austin's presence. Mom and dad were at a VIP party that was the next room over with breakfast foods and lots of door prizes. I saw the Orange Juice server. Not as big this time, but enough for a small party. I felt Austin's presence next to me, and then, when he was called to join the VIP section, I felt him getting up and leaving. I thought he had also kissed me first before going to the party.

## Half a year done, Lifetime to go

What a weird/interesting half-a-year it has been. I write letters now to my donor and their family so they learn a little about me and what it has been like sharing a heart.

A new pet peeve I have is a nurse or doctor saying

"Your heart looks great," or "Your heart is _____X, Y OR Z_____"

I know it shouldn't bother me, but right now, it does. While yes, it is my heart, the one I was born with is no longer here. Papa God is holding it. It is my borrowed heart.

## Seven months finished

It is weird waiting for a year to come around. I want to see so badly if my donor's family is willing to write or meet. I hope they will want to also. I finally saw my church family last Sunday. There was a potluck dinner with the Super Bowl on the big screen. I rolled in, and my pastor announced I was there and called me a celebrity. People who had heard my story but did not know me could now put a face to the name, and the people who have known us also came up and said hello while giving me hugs. I will hug just about anybody that I know, or I have not seen in awhile. My Ejection Fraction, or EF, has gone back five percent since the hospital as well. This is a good thing. The higher the number, the better the chance of the doctors letting hubby and I add to the family. Now, Mom and I are starting this Sunday, Feb 19th 2023. We are going to the churches we know that have been praying for me so people can see their prayers working.

## Ten Months later

May 2nd, 2023, I walked for the first time in months. **On** May 9th, I let women watch me walk. On May 11th, my heart turned 10 months old. May has been a very tricky month this year. Two weekends in a row, going to the same Emergency Department. The first time, they sent me home because the X-rays showed nothing. I had thought about my foot for sure being broken. But because of all the color, nothing showed up in any of the pictures. The following weekend, my hemoglobin was low, and where I had dialysis, I suggested I go back to the ED. I had no symptoms of my hemoglobin being low. But my foot was still a 10 out of 10 at times. After a few tests and letting out my frustrations, I finally got my answer. I ended up getting a baker's cyst sitting in between a vein and my calf muscle. Not only had it probably been there awhile, but it burst and bled. Bleeding all down my leg inside. My INR (how they measure how quickly my blood clots and how thin or thick it is) was way too high at 10! My normal range is 2-3. The Emergency Department gave me stuff to fight it, it was re-checked, and then without eating anything or moving it came back ten and a half! This was now past midnight, so they admitted me. Doctors kept giving me stuff to bring my INR down. By the time my room was ready, my INR had come down to a safer number to be moved. Let's see, I'm still here. I'm currently still in this stay. It is Thursday. Doctors want to do a heart Catheterization before I go home. It has almost been a year since the transplant, and while I'm here, they want to get those yearly tests out of the way. I have not been able to eat anything since midnight. I have so much on my mind and so many people I have questions for. My foot is in so much pain.

The catheterization went well. I fell asleep and felt nothing surprising. No heart disease or heart rejection! In recovery, I got too much blood clotting up. I ended up spending the night in ICU. They got the clot out, but with all the pressure on my hip, my entire hip from left to right turned black and blue now, just like my foot. But because there was a lot of blood lost, they gave me more blood through my IV.

So now, at times, my hips down to my feet hurt really bad. I still can't feel my feet. The times I do stand, it feels weird because my feet seem to go even more numb.

## Hello June

It's now June. I am still in the hospital. My heart will be eleven months old in a few weeks. My birthday is also coming up. My dream for this birthday is to walk on the beach, find a spot to lie down, listen to the waves, and feel the breeze. So, while here in the hospital, that is what my mind is going to be thinking about.

We are currently still waiting for my INR to go up. My weight keeps changing because no one wakes me up to take stuff off my bed. So now they want a standing weight every morning, and I can't stand by myself. So I am scared. I have a machine that helps me stand, but now, because of my big bruise on my hips, my legs will not straighten out for a standing weight. I have not taken a step. I am scared of falling.

I honestly had a hard time looking up to Christ. But I found a study on my Bible app that led me to a verse, and I drew what I saw.

The verse: 2 Corinthians chapter four verse seven.

But we have this treasure in jars of clay to show that this all-surpassing power is from God and not from us.

# June 2nd - A hard Day I can't forget.

Not having any of my journals here to write down what I am learning this stay is difficult; what I have accomplished here. But I do have this, my book, and here I can write down my thoughts in real-time. I woke up angry today. My Nurse practitioner wanted a standing weight this AM. Was she crazy? I've never stood up without my braces. My braces are back home. Also, the way she asked if someone could bring them rubbed me off the wrong way. No, my parents are two and a half hours away, and my husband is an hour and a half away and is working now. Today I felt lonely. So, I requested a pastoral-type person to talk to. I told her I keep trying to tell myself I am where God wants me to be, but when I talk it out to others, they all say something along the lines of how I've been set back. Then I start to question God: why am I set back while fighting my brain? I'm not set back at all. I am where God wants me to be. But yes, it is all very frustrating. I had no desire to call my husband today because he was going to work, and I was sad and upset, so I didn't want that to rub off on him for his night work. Well, my soul wanted him, and I couldn't fight it anymore. I video-called him, and he answered! I told him I was tired from dialysis and I was just not having a good day. God gave him the answer I needed. He had no idea either. Anyway, I told him I was mad because I stood without my braces long enough to get weighed this morning. His reaction this time was the reaction I wanted throughout this healing process. The reaction I wanted from the little steps I had been taking.

"Babe, this is absolutely amazing! Don't you see? You stood up to your best ability with very little assistance! This is huge, and I'm proud of you!"

You see, he saw what I failed to see. God is still moving and giving me the strength to get up and hold myself up.

PPhilippians 4:13: I can do all things through Christ who gives me strength.

So, I am continuing to study and write things down. Today's big takeaway is this: Not just being fixed is painful, but so is growing. My encouragement for today would be 1st Thessalonians chapter five, first half of verse twenty-three.

May God himself, the God of peace, sanctify you through and through.

As I try to look at things more positively today, I am super proud of how far I've come. I stood today, I did dialysis today, and I did a little stretch with physical therapy. Working on my ankles and feet, stretching them, felt good and hurt. Became tollable for me to keep going. I ended up coming home on June 7th.

My birthday is in the second week of June. I was very happy when I got to leave the hospital before my birthday and be home with my family for my birthday. This year, my brother and my husband came to where I am to celebrate with me. I got chocolates and sweet and sour candies. I got two purple shirts that I had shown the family I wanted for Christmas. One of my favorites was a notebook that I could write on and later erase. But the best part is taking a picture of my writing, and it goes into my computer where I tell it too. Being in a wheelchair makes it harder for my family to go out and do things, so we do what we can. But I dream of a day I can be able to do stuff I want to do, like walk on the beach.

## July - Finally here!

In July 2022, I was in the hospital, praying to God that I will be able to see July 2023. July of 2023 is finally here. On Tuesday July 11th, 2023, my mom and I, along with some deep family friends, celebrated my heart being a year old. The restaurant that we wanted to go to was closed for the day. Instead of canceling on us, Our friends invited us over to their house. We had sandwiches, blueberries, cherries, and a beautiful salad with a refreshing lemonade (If I am offered lemonade, I almost can not resist a cold one). Today, not only did we thank God for the gift of life for me, but we prayed for my donor's family. I see my transplant team again soon, and I am praying that my donor's family would love to meet me and hear my story. How their family members' heart, a heart they love, is someone else's first fully functioning heart!

The story I mentioned from the bible about Jesus washing his disciples' feet does not end with his death. NO! Three days later, he rose again! He even appeared to a few disciples to prove it! He did this because he loves us. Humanity. He wanted us to be able to meet with him and see HIM one day.

John 3:16 says for God so loved the world that he gave us his one and only son that whoever believes in him will not perish but have everlasting life.

Papa God, meets you where you are in life. He wants a relationship with you! You do not need to change for him, but he WILL change you.

The things you are doing now, that bad habit, will stop as you continue to grow and learn about Jesus. You are going to want to stop and make a change, and that is the beginning of God changing you and making you who HE wants you to be. HIS. His child forever and always!

Are you ready for that change? Ready for Papa God to start moving in your life? Maybe ready to come back to him and start over?

Here is a simple prayer yet powerful. He will listen and come.

Dear Papa God,

I am ready to have a relationship with you. I am ready to become your friend. I do believe that you, Jesus, died on the cross but rose on the third day! Thank you for thinking of me up on that cross as you did die for me. I believe it! Please come make my heart Jesus your home. I love you. In Jesus' name, Amen!

# Dear Family of my Donor...

To: The Family who loved my heart first,

Thank you times a MILLION and ONE PLUS. Thank you for choosing to give life through loss. I have been praying for you all since my doctor came into my ICU room and told me they had accepted a heart for me. The biggest thing I would want to tell you in person is your loved one's heart is my first ever fully functioning heart. The second thing I would want to tell you in person is I think about you guys and pray for you guys pretty much daily. The third and final thing I would want to tell you in person would be I already know of several people who became organ donors because your family gave and they heard my story of life. Thank you for loving and taking care of my heart.

www.ingramcontent.com/pod-product-compliance
Lightning Source LLC
Chambersburg PA
CBHW051249020426
42333CB00025B/3126